50 THINGS TO KNOW
BOOK SERIES
REVIEWS FROM READERS

I recently downloaded a couple of books from this series to read over the weekend thinking I would read just one or two. However, I so loved the books that I read all the six books I had downloaded in one go and ended up downloading a few more today. Written by different authors, the books offer practical advice on how you can perform or achieve certain goals in life, which in this case is how to have a better life.

The information is simple to digest and learn from, and is incredibly useful. There are also resources listed at the end of the book that you can use to get more information.

50 Things To Know To Have A Better Life: Self-Improvement Made Easy! by Dannii Cohen

---

This book is very helpful and provides simple tips on how to improve your everyday life. I found it to be useful in improving my overall attitude.

50 Things to Know For Your Mindfulness & Meditation Journey by Nina Edmondso

---

Quick read with 50 short and easy tips for what to think about before starting to homeschool.

50 Things to Know About Getting Started with Homeschool by Amanda Walton

I really enjoyed the voice of the narrator, she speaks in a soothing tone. The book is a really great reminder of things we might have known we could do during stressful times, but forgot over the years.

- HarmonyHawaii

50 Things to Know to Manage Your Stress: Relieve The Pressure and Return The Joy To Your Life

by Diane Whitbeck

There is so much waste in our society today. Everyone should be forced to read this book. I know I am passing it on to my family.

50 Things to Know to Downsize Your Life: How To Downsize, Organize, And Get Back to Basics

by Lisa Rusczyk Ed. D.

Great book to get you motivated and understand why you may be losing motivation. Great for that person who wants to start getting healthy, or just for you when you need motivation while having an established workout routine.

50 Things To Know To Stick With A Workout: Motivational Tips To Start The New You Today

by Sarah Hughes

50 THINGS TO KNOW ABOUT YOGA

Cover Image: https://pixabay.com/photos/yoga-girl-beach-sunset-summer-1665173/
Yoga Image 1: https://pixabay.com/photos/people-woman-yoga-meditation-2573216/
Yoga Image 2: https://pixabay.com/photos/yoga-woman-nature-landscape-1812695/
Yoga Image 3: https://pixabay.com/photos/poppies-yoga-field-woman-the-path-3644060/
Yoga Image 4: https://pixabay.com/photos/people-woman-pink-yoga-mat-2562216/

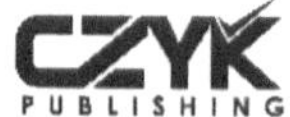

CZYK Publishing Since 2011.

50 Things to Know
Visit our website at www.50thingstoknow..com

Lock Haven, PA
All rights reserved.
ISBN: 9781793056535

50 THINGS TO KNOW ABOUT YOGA

BOOK DESCRIPTION

Do you want to try some yoga poses? Would you like to know what all things you'll need to attend a yoga class? Are you excited to learn which yoga style is right for you?

If you answered yes to any of these questions, then this 50 Things To Know book is for you.

50 Things To Know About Yoga by Sushmita Choudhury offers the answers to the most burning questions in yoga. Most books on yoga dive straight into the yoga poses. Although there's nothing wrong with that, this book will get down to the nitty-gritty of yoga that is often overlooked. Based on first-hand knowledge earned from teaching yoga to hundreds of students, this book will provide the much-needed guidance to yoga beginners.

In these pages, you'll discover actionable advice that will help you to make better, informed decisions in each step of your yoga journey. Before starting anything new, all you need is a little push and this book will give you just that and more. It will allow you to embrace yoga wholeheartedly.

By the time you finish this book, you'll have a clear understanding of yoga and what you can do to improve your yoga experience. So grab YOUR copy today. You'll be glad you did.

TABLE OF CONTENTS

13. Pay Attention To What Your Body Says
14. Avoid Comparisons
15. Communicate With Your Teacher
16. Reconsider Before Quitting
17. Hatha Yoga
18. Iyengar Yoga
19. Kundalini Yoga
20. Ashtanga Yoga
21. Hot Yoga
22. Yin Yoga
23. Restorative Yoga
24. Vinyasa Yoga
25. Prenatal Yoga

Beginner-Friendly Yoga Poses
26. Tadasana
27. Uttanasana
28. Dandasana
29. Virabhadrasana
30. Paschimottanasana
31. Pawanmuktasana
32. Trikonasana
33. Adho Mukha Svanasana
34. Vrikshasana
35. Bhujangasana
36. Marjariasana & Bitilasana

ABOUT THE AUTHOR

Sushmita Choudhury is a certified yoga trainer and a fitness expert. She fell in love with yoga after it cured her back pain. She now helps her students realize the benefits of practicing yoga. When she is not doing yoga, she likes to write. Also, she loves to draw, cook and watch movies.

INTRODUCTION

"The nature of yoga is to shine the light of awareness into the darkest corners of the body."

– Jason Crandell

Practicing yoga makes your body, mind and soul feel healthier. For starters, yoga helps to treat stress, anxiety, depression, headache, carpal tunnel syndrome, high and low blood pressure, arthritis, back pain, asthma, diabetes, heart problems and other diseases. It also helps to tone your muscles and reduce body fat. It increases your flexibility and stamina, enhances your blood circulation and strengthens your immune system. In a nutshell, yoga makes you feel better about yourself, boosts your self-esteem and teaches you to be confident in your own skin.

But this is just the beginning. The actual purpose of yoga lies deeper. Yoga is essentially a Sanskrit term. It originates from the root word "yuj" which means "to join". According to yogis, yoga was developed to connect the human body with the human mind and spirit. The last stage of yoga is enlightenment, attaining "Moksha" or liberation from the cycle of birth and death and becoming one with the divine consciousness. It's a journey that brings about inner peace and connects us with our surroundings. This is the reason why many yoga asanas take inspiration from the members of the plant or animal kingdom.

Yoga is thus a way of life. It leads you on a path of honesty and makes you a humble person. It teaches you to be in control of yourself. The best part about yoga is that it gives you the freedom to choose. So if you're someone who only wants to focus on physical well-being, you're totally allowed to do that. You can go about practicing your daily yoga routine without even bothering about the spiritual aspect of yoga and nobody will stop you. For whatever reason you decide to do yoga, yoga will definitely make you feel good about yourself.

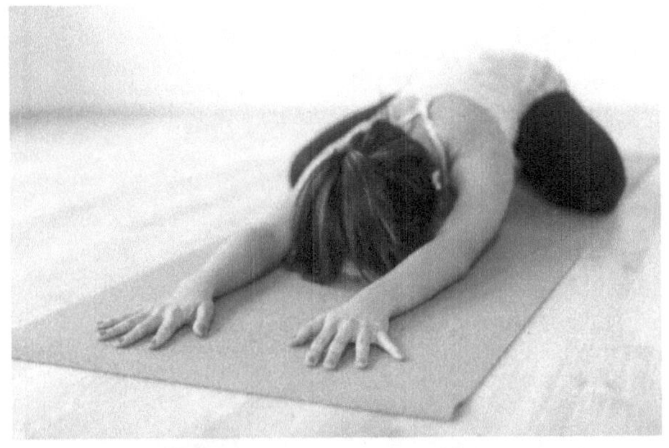

LET'S START WITH THE BASICS!

Now, that you're ready to begin your yoga journey, you must be wondering what all things you'll need to attend your yoga classes and if there are certain rules/norms that you must follow. Yes, there are; but they're also very doable!

Whether you join a yoga course at a yoga studio or decide to hire a personal yoga instructor, follow these few basic tips. By using this knowledge, you'll feel even more confident about your decision and will be fully prepared to attend any yoga class.

1. CHOOSING THE RIGHT CLOTHES FOR YOGA

Clothes form an important aspect of our lives. Right clothes make us feel in-charge.

Your clothes should be such that they complement your activities. When choosing your yoga outfit, always go for the comfortable and slightly loose ones. Since yoga involves a ton of bending and stretching moves, wearing loose-fitting outfits will allow all your joints, and thus your entire body to move freely and easily. Trust me, this comes in very handy. Wearing loose-fitting, breathable clothes will ensure that there is proper air circulation throughout the body while working out.

Since yoga also involves bending postures, ensure that your garments are tight enough that they don't slide down when you bend over. Who wants to put themselves in an embarrassing situation in front of their teacher, right? Finally, if you're feeling cold, put on a jumper. Just remember, the jumper should also allow free body movement. Simple. Now on to the next tip.

2. YOGA SOCKS AND GLOVES

Consider investing in a good pair of yoga socks and gloves. Whether it's the winter months or maybe your limbs are cold from the air conditioning in the room, these gloves and socks will definitely provide the much-needed warmth so that you can be mentally and physically present while practicing yoga.

One of the other important function of the yoga gloves or the yoga socks is to provide some extra traction. Being specifically designed to cling to your yoga mat or other surfaces like the floor or carpet, the gloves or socks will prevent you from slipping during your yoga practice. Yoga gloves, being ergonomically formulated, will also provide extra support in doing yoga poses that put pressure on your wrists like the downward facing dog pose, plank etc.

Owing to their non-slippery property, the yoga gloves and socks are also a great alternative to the traditional travel yoga mats. This makes them incredibly useful if you're someone who loves to travel. Also, they take up less space in your bags as compared to mats.

Apart from all these benefits, just like normal socks and gloves, yoga socks and gloves are also hygienic. They help to protect your hands and feet from coming in direct contact with dust particles and germs.

3. CHOOSING THE RIGHT ACCESSORIES AND PROPS

In order to continue with any yoga routine, there are a few basic yoga props and accessories that you will require. These are the yoga mat, yoga straps, yoga blocks, and yoga blankets. It is advisable to start with the cheap options first. Later depending on the type of yoga you choose, you can invest in the right accessories.

Yoga mats and blankets provide a non-slippery surface so that you can accurately do your yoga poses, whereas yoga straps and blocks help you to stretch and twist your body a little more. Apart from this, yoga props also provide extra support, help to increase flexibility and aid in correct alignment of the body.

Before buying your own props, you can also check if your yoga studio offers these on rent. It is a great way to understand your needs and also save a few bucks!

4. EATING BEFORE PRACTICE

As you ease into your yoga routine, you'll find yourself doing tons of body twisting movements and flowing from one yoga pose to another. While this might sound intimidating at first, just remember to trust your instructor. They will help you through all of it. But there is one other way to help yourself do all those movements with considerable ease - that is by eating on time.

If you attend your yoga classes on a full stomach or a stomach that is trying to digest something heavy, it'll make you feel very uncomfortable. Ideally, you must eat two to four hours before your workout. But if you fear you'll start starving, you can eat a light meal an hour before class or have a banana at least 20 minutes before practice.

In order to make the most of your yoga classes, ensure that your bowels and stomach are empty before you start your workout.

5. ARRIVING EARLY

There are primarily two ways to learn yoga - one is with the help of a personal instructor who will guide you on a one-to-one basis and the other route is to join a yoga studio. If you've decided to take the latter path, then this particular tip is for you.

On your first day, reach your studio at least 20 minutes before your class starts. As a new student, this will give you some time to fill out any paperwork or to ask about the workout schedule or to know if the studio offers any discounts.

Also, you can utilize this time to introduce yourself to your teacher. Try talking to some of the other students and let them know that you're a beginner. This will boost your confidence.

6. KEEP YOUR SHOES OUTSIDE

Shoes should be left on the rack while practicing yoga. You'll notice that this will help you to balance yourself while doing the various yoga poses. Also, it will help you to connect with yourself and your surroundings and make you feel grounded.

7. YOUR PHONE SHOULD BE IN YOUR BAG

Though it's true that smartphones have become an inseparable part of our lives, you should keep your phone aside during your yoga classes.

If you're someone who keeps checking their phone now and then, this step is a must. Switch off the phone and put it in your bag. If you keep using your phone during the classes, not only will this prevent you from concentrating on your routine, it will also disturb others around you.

8. PRACTICE, PRACTICE, PRACTICE!

*"The very heart of yoga practice
is 'abyhasa' – steady effort in the
direction you want to go."*

– Sally Kempton

It takes time to become good at something. Same is the case with yoga. There will be days when the yoga studio is closed or your personal yoga teacher is on leave. On those days, it will entirely be on you to practice.

Instead of being lazy, lay out your yoga mat and get going. Do what your teacher has taught. Just remember to follow the exact instructions. You can also ask your instructor about anything specific that you should keep in mind while practicing yoga on your own.

Make it a habit to practice yoga every day. Do it in short sessions, if you want. Develop a routine that you're comfortable with, a routine that can grow with you. You'll surely notice a positive change in your life as you develop a regular habit to practice yoga.

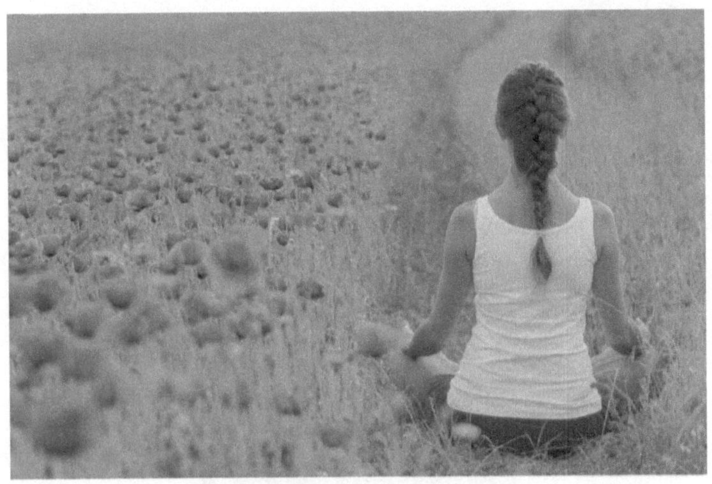

WHILE IN CLASS

Yoga serves as a means of joining the body, mind and individual spirit with the spirit of God. In order to reap the full benefits of yoga, you'll have to learn to be present in the moment.

The following points will guide you through this. Also, you'll get to know what you should expect from a typical yoga class.

9. EMBRACE YOURSELF

*"Yoga is the journey of the self,
through the self, to the self."*

– The Bhagavad Gita

Yoga gives you an opportunity to connect with your inner self. Use this time judiciously to introspect. You'll notice that your understanding of your body and mind has improved.

Even though this might sound a little selfish, but while doing yoga just focus on yourself, your wants, your regrets. Concentrate on yourself as a person and embrace your true self.

10. CHANTING

As per Yogapedia, chanting is defined as "a rhythmical repetition (either silently or aloud) of a song, prayer, word or sound. It is one of the most ancient spiritual practices and a part of most religions and spiritual paths."

Chanting, in yoga, mainly involves repeating Sanskrit mantras. Depending on your yoga studio, chanting might be done at the beginning or towards the end of the class.

It's completely up to you to decide if you want to incorporate chanting in your daily yoga regimen. But if you do decide to give chanting a go, ask your teacher or the studio if they can provide a written version of the chant so that it's easy for you to memorize. Then during your practice, try to repeat it with everybody else in the class.

While chanting, it's alright if you make a mistake here and there. Everyone does at their initial stages. But what's more important is to relax and to keep an open mind. You'll slowly notice that by introducing chanting in your yoga routine, all those negative thoughts inside your head have reduced. Thus your mind will become calmer and this will bring in a sense of inner peace.

11. LEARN TO RELAX

As a yoga beginner, you might notice that while doing a pose/asana you're clenching your jaws, fingers, and toes or maybe holding your breath. These reactions are actually a physical representation of the stress that your body and mind are going through while doing the yoga pose. This happens because we have become conditioned to take stress whenever we have to deal with a situation that takes us out of our comfort zones.

In order to mitigate this stress, you'll have to learn to relax. The ability to stay calm during stressful times is an immensely important, yet overlooked aspect of our lives. Relaxation reduces anxiety and improves our overall health. Being able to relax comes with time. A quick way to start practicing relaxation is during your yoga classes.

While doing any yoga asana, focus on your breath. Once you start doing this, you'll feel more comfortable and will also be able to maintain your poses for longer durations. Just by concentrating on your breath, you'll have the power to let go of all that stress and finally relax. Now let's discuss about breathing in a little more detail.

12. BREATHING

"Inhale the future. Exhale the past."

– Anonymous

Yoga ceases to be yoga without proper breathing. When your yoga teacher instructs you to focus on your breathing, what they actually mean is to become aware of your inhalations and exhalations, that means, your breathing cycle. Once you become aware of your breathing cycle, you can then move on to the next step, which is knowing when to inhale and when to exhale during any particular yoga posture.

Before discussing that, let us briefly talk about how our body's anatomy changes when we breathe. When you inhale, your belly expands outward and your chest moves upward and outward, thereby expanding your front body. The exact opposite happens when you exhale and the front portion of your body tends to collapse inward.

Thus body movement and breath are inherently connected. All yoga postures intelligently utilize this link. Based on this link, there are two basic guidelines of breathing that should be followed while doing any yoga pose.

In any asana, where you open or extend your front body, you must inhale. This includes movements such as backbends, raising your arms.

In any asana, where you compress your front body, you must exhale. This includes movements such as forward bends, twists or side bends.

By following these two rules, your body will relax and you'll be able to hold poses for longer durations. Also, by focusing on your breath, your mind will stay focused, which will allow you to stay present in the moment on your yoga mat. If you ever find your mind wandering, lengthen the inhales and exhales. It will help you to calm down and return to your practice with a fresh mindset.

13. PAY ATTENTION TO WHAT YOUR BODY SAYS

While doing a pose, if your breath becomes restricted, then you should stop right there. Being unable to breathe during an asana is an indication that your body has been pushed in such a way that will do more harm than good. Also, refrain from doing a yoga posture that is causing pain in your body.

Every pose in yoga can be modified to suit a student's requirements. Consult your instructor to devise a routine that meets your needs and physique. During practicing any asana, if your body says no, even for once, listen to it immediately. Stop doing that asana and inform your teacher. On the contrary, if you continue with the asana, your body will be under constant tension and your breathing will be adversely affected, which will not only defeat the purpose of yoga but can also lead to injuries.

The goal of yoga is to make you feel relaxed and good about yourself. In order for that to happen, there has to be a proper balance between breathing and movement. Once you strike this balance, throughout your session, you'll be able to take long, deep breaths, move your body and hold your poses effortlessly. Only then will you derive the true benefit of yoga.

14. AVOID COMPARISONS

"A flower does not think of competing to the flower next to it. It just blooms."

– Zen Shin

Needless to say, any kind of comparison only makes us feel even more miserable about ourselves. Still, why do we compare? It's because, from childhood, we become conditioned to compare ourselves with friends, cousins and as we grow up, unbeknownst to us, this comparison becomes a deeply ingrained habit.

But, it's crucial to understand that by comparing ourselves with others around us, we're wasting our own time and energy. This habit of comparison just makes us less productive and takes us farther away from our goals and dreams.

So, during your yoga sessions, refrain from comparing yourself with the other practitioners. Instead, focus on your own capabilities. There must be some reason as to why you started learning yoga in the first place. Remind yourself of that goal, so that inferiority complex can't stop you.

Unless you're learning yoga on a one-to-one basis, you'll see that in any yoga class there are students of varied age groups and fitness levels. They're all unique in their own ways, just like you, hence any kind of comparison would be unfitting on everybody's part.

Yoga is anything but a competitive workout session, where everybody is trying to look their best and show off their strength and flexibility. The absence of mirrors in yoga studios further reinstates this point. Without mirrors, there remains no way for the students to know how they're looking while doing a particular pose. This actually has two main advantages. Firstly, this reduces comparisons with the other students. Secondly, the students learn to trust their teacher and most importantly, their own instincts. They're then able to shift their focus from how they look to how they feel during the stretches, which finally enables them to connect to their true selves.

Thus yoga is a therapy that helps you to break free of all kinds of physical and emotional inhibitions that are holding you back. Therefore, whenever you practice yoga, listen to your teacher, concentrate on the movements of your body, concentrate on your breathing and in the process, try to become fully aware of each and every sensation you experience.

15. COMMUNICATE WITH YOUR TEACHER

"A photographer gets people to pose for him. A yoga instructor gets people to pose for themselves."

– T. Guillemets

Your yoga teacher is your "friend, philosopher and guide". You must clearly communicate with him/her regarding any problem you face during your sessions.

During the starting days, you may find that the classes are paced a little too fast or maybe too slow and you're having trouble keeping up with the rest of the students. Understand that this happens with many starters. You need to have patience and follow the directions given to you. But if you find that this is affecting your self-confidence, do talk to your teacher. As your mentor, she/he will definitely help you out.

If you have suffered from any physical ailments and injuries recently or maybe in the past, this is also something that your instructor must know. In fact, your instructor must know about it from the first day itself. Health issues like heart problems, back pain, high blood pressure are contraindicative. Hence having prior knowledge about your health is critical in order for your trainer to modify the asanas so that you can derive the maximum benefit from yoga.

Sometimes sudden body stretches can lead to muscle cramps. Some students even report feeling dizzy or experiencing headaches after a long workout. This predominantly happens in the case of those students who mostly lead a sedentary life. If you're someone who is experiencing such symptoms, definitely let your teacher know.

Your yoga teacher is a vital part of your yoga journey. In order to minimize the risk of any kind of injury and to have a safe training, it's important that you practice yoga as per his/her directions.

16. RECONSIDER BEFORE QUITTING

It happens with many students that after joining a yoga class, within a couple of days they feel disappointed. They decide to quit as they start believing yoga is not for them.

But this is far from the truth. Yoga has something for everybody. These students fail to realize that their chosen style of yoga and/or their chosen yoga studio is the actual culprit; and not yoga in general.

If you ever find yourself in the same situation, consider trying out other options before deciding to quit. If you like an intense workout, then you could explore Hot Yoga, Vinyasa Yoga or Ashtanga Yoga.

On the other hand, if you like something slow sailing, Kundalini Yoga, Yin or Iyengar Yoga might be the right one for you. Irrespective of your choice, all of these yoga styles will provide similar benefits.

Also, consider evaluating if you're able to understand and follow your yoga instructor. An experienced yoga instructor is a must to lead the way and guide you on your yoga journey. Many yoga studios and personal yoga teachers offer demo classes. Consider enrolling yourself in these classes to give few of them a try. This will give you enough exposure to find your favorite yoga studio, teacher and style of yoga.

It's okay if you find that you prefer one trainer over another or one form of yoga over another form of yoga. But what's more important is to never give up on yoga. Yoga is an all-inclusive practice. With all its possible modifications, yoga is so diverse that anybody can find a style that speaks to them.

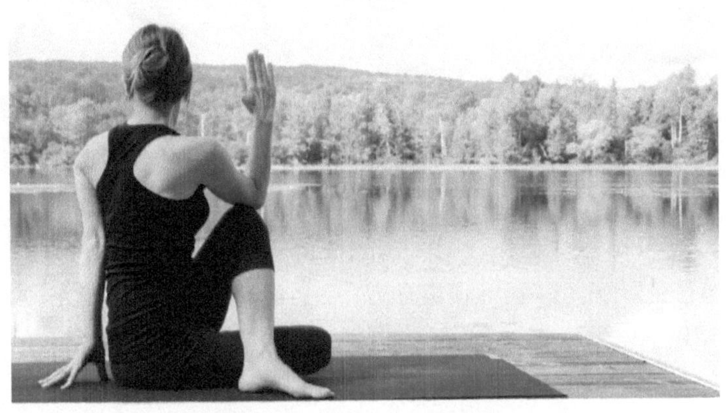

STYLES OF YOGA

Choosing one's favorite style of yoga is easier said than done. It's usually seen that depending on your present situation like age, health, a particular kind of yoga will resonate more in comparison to others. This might change as your circumstances change and you could find yourself getting drawn to the other styles.

But, in order to get the ball rolling, you have to zero in on one particular yoga technique that you can relate to the most in your current state of mind. So how do you do that? Well, the only reliable way is by trying out a couple of different types of yoga, in person.

Let's discuss nine different forms of yoga that are widely practiced by various yogis around the world. All of these fall under two broad categories - rigorous and gentle. While going through these, ask yourself what kind of yoga practice are you looking for? Do you want something sweaty and athletic or should it have a more lenient approach? Irrespective of what you choose, make it a point to attend your classes with an open mind and to stick to your choice for a considerable amount of time, to completely understand if it works for you.

17. HATHA YOGA

"Hatha" is a Sanskrit word that translates to "force" or "forceful". So, hatha yoga is a form of yoga that incorporates physical movements as a way to balance the body and mind.

It is one of the six original types of yoga, along with Karma Yoga, Raja Yoga, Gyana Yoga, Bhakti Yoga, and Mantra Yoga. Hatha Yoga, in its raw form, includes cleansing techniques such as pranayama, mudras/gestures, meditation, asanas, and shat kriyas. But in present times, the focus has mainly shifted to practicing asanas and concentrating on your breathing.

A typical hatha yoga class is slow paced. Students are asked to perform some fundamental yoga postures that will improve their flexibility. Each posture is held for a certain number of breaths. This brings in a sense of calmness and prepares the students for meditation and pranayama.

Hatha yoga is one of the gentler forms of yoga. It is best suited for people who want to feel relaxed yet stretched out after their yoga session. With its classic approach to exercising and breathing, it is a great option for beginners who want a clearer understanding of yoga in general.

Over the years, many styles of yoga have originated from hatha yoga. The following eight styles are some of those. The relation of hatha yoga with the other styles is that of a parent and child. Each of the styles is similar to hatha yoga in some aspect, yet have their own distinct characteristics that appeal to a specific group of yoga aspirants.

18. IYENGAR YOGA

Iyengar yoga was established by B.K.S Iyengar. This is a detail-oriented form of yoga.

Iyengar students practice yoga with an emphasis on proper alignment of the body while doing the yoga asanas. Along with alignment, another important aspect of Iyengar yoga is that once you attain the desired form of a pose, you'll have to hold it for a long time. In order to achieve this, students focus on controlling their breathing and using yoga props like blankets, straps, blocks, bolsters, etc.

Iyengar yoga is definitely beginner-friendly. By combining breathing and props, it helps you to increase your flexibility, in a safe yet effective manner. Since Iyengar teachers undergo comprehensive trainings, they possess invaluable knowledge about human anatomy and movement, which they generously share in their classes.

Also, Iyengar yoga can be practiced by people of all age groups. Due to its slow, controlled and methodical approach, it is great for those who want to overcome chronic health conditions and injuries.

19. KUNDALINI YOGA

According to ancient Hindu scriptures, "Kundalini", also known as kundalini energy is a type of primal spiritual energy, pictured as a coiled serpent, that is said to exist at the base of our spinal cords. Kundalini yoga aims to release this energy so that you can rise above your internal conflicts and reach an advanced stage of self-awareness.

Kundalini yoga classes are physically and mentally challenging. Students perform "kriyas" in which they repeatedly practice a set of restorative asanas along with intense breathing. Apart from physical exercises and breath work, students also practice mantra chanting, bandha, pranayama, and meditation.

With such a wide array of activities, Kundalini yoga is one of the most comprehensive forms of yoga. If you're looking for a yoga form that is intense, yet strikes a balance between physical and spiritual upliftment, then Kundalini yoga is the one for you.

20. ASHTANGA YOGA

"Asht" means "eight" and "anga" means "parts/components". So, the Sanskrit word "Ashtanga" means "having eight components/parts" and Ashtanga yoga refers to a type of yoga that has eight parts. But, nowadays, most yoga studios focus on only one part, and that is practicing asanas.

This style of yoga is intensive and systematic. Students practice specific asanas in the exact same order in each class and synchronize their movements with their breath. The asanas that are chosen are physically taxing and generate body heat, that leads to sweating.

Ashtanga yoga is suited for those who are used to vigorous workouts. So if you're someone who does gym and is already active, you can attempt Ashtanga and see if it works out for you. Apart from this, since Ashtanga follows a set approach to yoga, predictability might also be a factor that draws you to try out this yoga form.

21. HOT YOGA

As the name suggests, Hot yoga is a yoga form that aims to achieve the benefits of yoga by practicing in a hot environment.

Yoga studios and teachers encourage students to do yoga in a heated room. The heat makes it easier for the students to stretch their bodies. As a result, their bodies work harder and this increases their heart rates. The intense workout coupled with the existing heat in the room causes profuse sweating. This sweating is said to detoxify the students' body and mind by flushing out toxins.

Hot yoga helps to develop body flexibility and core strength, like cardiovascular workouts. If you love strict workout routines that leave you soaked in sweat, then sign up for a hot yoga class designed for beginners. Just remember to drink sufficient amount of water before, during and after your class to protect yourself from dehydration.

22. YIN YOGA

Yin classes helps students go deeper into yoga. In Yin yoga, students hold a particular yoga pose for 3 - 5 minutes. This intensifies their workout. Also, this lets the students access their body tissues and bones, rather than just their muscles.

Yin yoga attempts to restore the mobility in your joints and tissues. It also restores the flow of energy or "prana" throughout your body. Holding a yoga pose for 5 minutes straight is challenging. If you are a non-gym goer and are looking for something that will make you feel the burn, then Yin yoga is the right fit for you.

23. RESTORATIVE YOGA

Some people confuse restorative yoga with yin yoga. Even though both these styles involve holding yoga asanas for several minutes, the main difference lies in the fact that restorative yoga focuses only on the relaxation aspect of yoga. The intense nature of yoga is absent.

The main goal of restorative yoga is to heal and restore your body to its normal functioning. If you have some injuries or have undergone surgeries, then you can try restorative yoga. Also, it is ideal for you if you want to do yoga just for relaxing your body and mind, without diving into the physical workout and spiritual sides of yoga.

24. VINYASA YOGA

The term "vinyasa" has two parts: "nyasa" which means "to place" and "vi" which means "a special manner". Combining these two, "vinyasa" means "to place something in a special manner".

In vinyasa yoga, the postures are sequenced so that you flow from one pose to another, all the while being aware of your breath. It's like doing a dance, in which you're constantly doing some sort of movement.

This is an adaptive style of yoga in which the yoga trainers are free to plan their own classes. So classes vary from one trainer to another. Teachers usually include some kind of upbeat music, with beats matching the yoga sequences to increase the energy level of the class.

Along with boosting flexibility, vinyasa yoga also helps to increase your stamina and strengthen your core muscles. This form of fast-paced yoga is perfect for athletes, runners and intense exercisers, who are looking for ways to burn some calories.

25. PRENATAL YOGA

Prenatal yoga is specifically designed to cater to pregnant women and new moms. It focuses on breathing and involves exercises that strengthen the lower back and the pelvic floor muscles. Yoga props like bolsters, blocks, and blankets further enhance the experience.

This type of yoga helps expectant mothers bond with their growing babies. It physically and emotionally supports them through their pregnancy and prepares them for their labor and delivery. New moms can continue prenatal yoga even after their delivery for postpartum fitness.

Thus prenatal yoga is ideal for women who want to continue doing yoga during different phases of their pregnancy.

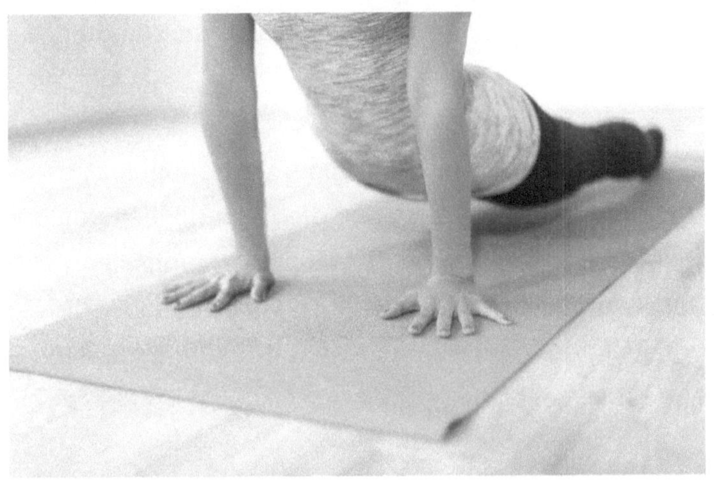

BEGINNER-FRIENDLY YOGA POSES

Each style of yoga has one thing in common, and that is the practice of asanas or yoga poses. Whether you choose slow-paced yoga or a fast-paced, intense form of yoga, asanas are the exercises that will help you to flex your muscles. Following is a list of eighteen different asanas that are useful for beginners.

26. TADASANA

"Tada" is a Sanskrit word that means "mountain". Thus Tadasana is also known as the Mountain Pose. It is the foundation pose for all asanas and is often seen as the 'mother of asanas'. Majority of the standing poses start from Tadasana.

Initially, this asana may seem very simple, as it just involves standing in one place. But, when you do it correctly, Tadasana will stretch every muscle in your body, challenge your consciousness and will connect you to your inner self spiritually, mentally and physically.

Tadasana has numerous benefits. It tones your abdomen, hips, and thighs. It strengthens your ankles and knees. It is great for relieving back pain. It also improves body posture and corrects flat feet.

One repetition of Tadasana takes around 10 - 20 seconds. To start, stand straight, with your feet slightly apart. Keep your hands along your body, hanging normally. Firm your thigh. Keep your lower belly muscles loose. Now slowly firm your inner ankles and lift them. Imagine energy is flowing through your ankles, thighs, spine, neck, reaching straight up to your head.

Keep breathing naturally. Slowly elongate your neck, so that you're now looking at the ceiling. Inhale and extend your chest and arms upwards. Hold your breath and lift your heels such that you are standing on your toes. You'll feel a stretch throughout your body. To further increase this stretch, you can interlock your fingers. Stay in the pose for 10 - 20 seconds. In order to release the pose, firstly exhale and then return to your starting position.

If you suffer from headaches or insomnia or have low blood pressure, consult your instructor for some modifications to this pose.

27. UTTANASANA

Uttanasana is also known as the Standing Forward Bend pose. It is a powerful stretching pose. In fact, the word "Ut" means "strong/powerful" and "tan" means "to pull/to stretch".

Uttanasana stretches your hamstrings, calves, back and hip muscles. This produces a profound relaxing sensation throughout the body that reduces stress and anxiety. This asana also helps to cure headache, insomnia, asthma, sinusitis, osteoporosis and high blood pressure. Apart from this, Uttanasana also contributes to the proper functioning of the digestive organs and kidneys and heals menstrual problems. If you have glaucoma, sciatica and/or suffer from lower back injury, you can give this asana a miss.

To do Uttanasana, stand on your mat like you would in Tadasana. Take a deep breath. Keep your knees loose. Exhale and slowly bend forward from your hips. Keep your hands on the mat beside your feet, such that they are parallel. As you bend further, you'll experience a pull in your hamstring muscles. Stay in the pose for as long as you want. When you're done, inhale and slowly raise your hands and upper body to stand up in the starting position.

28. DANDASANA

The Sanskrit word "Danda" means "stick". So Dandasana is called the Staff Pose in English. Like

Tadasana, this pose might also seem very plain at first, but with time you'll start appreciating its benefits. Practicing Dandasana will correct your posture and strengthen your muscles. It will increase your concentration power and reduce stress. Also, if you're suffering from asthma or sciatica, this asana will help to cure them.

To practice Dandasana, sit straight on your yoga mat and stretch out your legs, placing them parallel to each other. Your crown should be towards the ceiling and you should be able to look straight. Keep breathing naturally. Now bend your toes towards yourself. Press your buttocks and your heels down on the floor. Next, put your palms beside your hips and ensure that they are lying flat on the floor. If you have long arms, you can slightly bend your arms at the elbows. Relax your shoulder and legs. Stay in this pose for about 20 - 30 seconds and then release.

It is important to sit straight in this pose. If you find yourself constantly slouching, use a wall as support. Also, you can take a blanket, fold it and keep it below your buttocks, to sit properly with your legs stretched. Lastly, for people with carpal tunnel syndrome, keep your palms on the floor and then turn your hands so that your fingers point to your back. This will allow your muscles to properly stretch.

29. VIRABHADRASANA

Virabhadrasana or Warrior pose is an elegant yoga posture. It tones the arms and legs. For people with desk jobs, this asana revitalizes the spine and the shoulders. It also provides a sense of grounding, peace and inner bliss.

To do Virabhadrasana, start by placing your feet about three to four feet apart. Turn the right foot by ninety degrees, making sure it points outwards. Also, align the heel of your right foot with your left foot's center. Inhale and raise your arms sideways to your shoulder height. Ensure that the arms are parallel to the ground and the palms face upwards.

Next, exhale. Bring your right knee and ankle in a straight line by bending the right knee. Continue breathing naturally. Slowly turn your head so that you're looking to your right. After this, raise your arms above your head and join your palms. Also, raise your head such that you can see your palms.

If you feel comfortable, you can try to increase the separation between your feet while standing in this position. This will produce a nice stretch. After holding the pose for 20 seconds, inhale and bring your feet to the starting position. Next, exhale and bring your arms to your sides. Repeat for another 20 seconds on your left side, with the left knee bent.

If you suffer from shoulder pains, keeping your arms extended at shoulder height will be enough. Just make sure that they are parallel to the floor. For knee pain and arthritis problems, use a wall as support while practicing the asana. If you're a heart patient or have high blood pressure, you can skip this asana.

30. PASCHIMOTTANASANA

Remember the Sanskrit term "Uttan" from Uttanasana. "Uttan" means to provide an intense stretch. When you combine "Uttan" with "Paschima", you get the term "Paschimottan". Now, "Paschima" literally translates to "West". But in ancient times, the back of the body was called "West" or "Paschima" (the front of the body was called "Purva" or "East").

So, Paschimottanasana is a yoga asana that stretches your back muscles. For this reason, it is also known as the Intense Dorsal Stretch in English. The other name of this asana is the Seated Forward Bend owing to the way it's done.

Paschimottanasana targets a number of body parts and organs like shoulders, spinal cord, thigh muscles, liver, kidney, ovaries, and the uterus. It is extremely beneficial for women post delivery. It cures headaches, anxiety, insomnia, blood pressure issues, improves digestion and reduces obesity.

To practice this asana, sit down on your yoga mat. Keep your spine straight. Extend your legs in front and point your toes towards you. Inhale and stretch your arms above your head. Exhale and bend forward from your hips. In this position, without over stretching, extend your arms as if you want to touch your toes with your fingers. Hold for 10 - 20 seconds. Inhale and slowly lift your upper body, with the arms outstretched. Finally, exhale, sit up straight and bring your hands down.

New moms should practice Paschimottanasana only after delivery. If you suffer from diarrhea and asthma, refrain from doing this asana. Also, if you have back pain, practice this pose under the supervision of your instructor.

31. PAWANMUKTASANA

Pawanmuktasana is called the Wind-Relieving Pose in English as "Pawan" means "wind" and "Mukta" means "to release or to relieve". The "wind" here refers to the digestive gases that are formed within the stomach and the intestines.

By releasing the trapped digestive gases, Pawanmuktasana helps in better digestion. It also massages the reproductive and digestive organs. This asana stretches the back and the neck regions and helps to strengthen the pelvic muscles, abdominal muscles and the back muscles. Additionally, it also tones the arms, legs, and hips by burning fat in those areas.

To practice Pawanmuktasana, lie down on your mat, with your face facing upwards. Keep your arms beside you. Join your feet. Now, inhale. As you start exhaling, fold your legs at the knees and bring them to your chest. Tightly hold your legs with your hands and press the thighs creating pressure on your abdomen.

Keep breathing normally. When you're comfortable, exhale and lift your neck so as to touch your forehead to your knees. During all the exhales, increase the pressure on your abdomen by little and during the inhales, loosen it a little, so as to maintain a balance. You can also roll three to four times if you want. When you're done, release the pose.

If you have neck pain, you can keep your head resting on the floor. Give this asana a miss if you're pregnant, have high blood pressure, back problems, piles, hernia, slip disc or have recently undergone any kind of abdominal surgeries.

32. TRIKONASANA

"Trikona" means "triangle". Thus Trikonasana is also called the Triangle Pose. Practicing Trikonasana is known to cure osteoporosis, neck pain, back pain, sciatica, flat feet. It stretches and strengthens the muscles in your shoulders, chest, back, hips, groins up to your hamstrings and calves. It also improves your digestive capabilities.

Trikonasana is done separately on each leg. Start with the right side. Stand in Virabhadrasana, with the heel of your right foot aligned with the arch of the left foot. Inhale. As you start exhaling, bend your upper body to your right. At the same time, slowly raise your left arm such that it is in a straight line with your right arm. If you feel comfortable, you can turn your head to look at your left palm.

Even though you can keep your right palm anywhere on the lower portion of your right leg, it's best if you can place your palm on the floor. Continue breathing normally. After holding for 10 - 20 seconds, slowly raise your upper body and stand in your starting position, with both arms resting on your sides. Repeat the same steps on your left side. Alternate between each leg, repeating 3 - 5 times on each.

Refrain from doing this asana if you have headaches or low blood pressure. If you have high blood pressure, look downwards and if you have neck issues, look straight.

33. ADHO MUKHA SVANASANA

The word "Adho" means "down", "Mukha" means "face" and "Svana" means "dog. So, Adho Mukha Svanasana translates to Downward Facing Dog Pose. It is named so because it mimics the way a dog stretches its body when it bends forward.

This asana elongates the spine and stretches the hamstrings. It tones your hands and legs. It improves blood circulation throughout the body. Adho Mukha Svanasana also works on the abdominal muscles and enhances digestion.

To do this asana, first stand on all four of your limbs, forming a table. Now you need to form an inverted V structure. For this, exhale and push your hips up towards the ceiling and straighten your knees and elbows. Adjust the distance between each of your hand and legs so that you can stay balanced and your joints are relaxed. Now slowly push your hands on the floor and look towards your navel. Stay in this position for 10 - 20 seconds and then release starting with your knees and elbows.

If you are pregnant or are suffering from high blood pressure, shoulder injuries, carpal tunnel syndrome or detached retina, do this pose only under the supervision of your yoga teacher. Also, if you find it difficult to bend over, use a wall as support. Stand three feet from a wall, facing it. Place your palms on the wall and straighten your elbow. Slowly bring your hands to your torso level, so that your arms become parallel to the ground.

34. VRIKSHASANA

Vrikshasana is called Tree Pose in English because "Vriksh" means "tree". It is an elegant pose. It helps to tone your arms and legs. It improves neuromuscular coordination. It also strengthens the spine, shoulder, and knees. This asana improves the health or your eyes and inner ears, thereby enhancing your concentration and balance.

To practice Vrikshasana, stand straight with arms by your side. Keep breathing normally. Slowly bend the right knee and place the sole of your right foot high on your left thigh. Look straight. Take a deep

breath, bring your arms above your head and join
your palms.

Ensure that your spine remains straight all along.
Hold for 50 - 60 seconds or as long as you can
balance. When you want to release the pose, exhale
and bring your arms back to your side. Finally, place
your right foot on the floor. Repeat with your left
foot. Do 5 such repetitions with each leg.

If you have high blood pressure, instead of taking
your arms above your head, hold them in front of
your chest and then join your palms. If you have been
diagnosed with migraine or insomnia, you can give
this asana a miss.

35. BHUJANGASANA

"Bhujanga" is the Sanskrit word for "cobra".
Bhujangasana or the Cobra Pose tries to replicate a
cobra's raised hood. This pose has numerous benefits.
It stretches the internal organs thereby improving the
functioning of the respiratory, digestive, urinary and
reproductive systems. This, in turn, enhances
metabolism. The Cobra Pose is great for those who

want to lose weight. It also helps to make the spine flexible.

To practice Bhujangasana, lie down on the stomach, with hands on your side and ensure that your legs are stretched out and your toes touch one another. Now bring your hand to your shoulder level with palms facing the floor. Inhale, put your body weight on your palms and slowly arch your neck towards your back as you raise your upper body from your hips. Keep breathing naturally. Stay in the pose for about 15 - 20 seconds. Then exhale and come back to the starting position.

If you are pregnant or have undergone abdominal surgeries in the recent past, give Bhujangasana a miss. Also, if you're suffering from back injuries, hernia, headache or carpal tunnel syndrome, refrain from doing this asana.

36. MARJARIASANA & BITILASANA

Marjariasana and Bitilasana comprise a popular combination pose in yoga. These two are done one after another, starting with the Bitilasana and completing with the Marjariasana. Marjariasana is called the Cat Pose ("Marjari" means "cat") and Bitilasana is called the Cow Pose ("Bitil" means "cow").

Both these asanas are stress relievers. They also stretch and improve the flexibility of the spinal cord. This helps cure back pain and sciatica. The asanas also improve blood circulation. Individually, the Cow Pose stretches the muscles in the chest and neck regions, while the Cat Pose boosts the functioning of the digestive organs. Additionally, the Cat Pose also helps to reduce belly fat.

To practice this combo pose, start by bending your knees and sit on all fours, that is both your hands and knees. Your back will now be like a table top. Keep your feet neutral. Make sure that your wrists are in line with your shoulders and your knees are in line with your hips.

Take a deep breath. Gently push your buttocks in an upward direction. You'll notice that automatically your abdomen moves downwards and your chest muscles feel stretched. Look up by bending your neck upwards. Stay in this position for 15 seconds while breathing normally. Then exhale and slowly return to your starting position. This was Bitilasana.

To move on to Marjariasana, exhale and start arching your back. At the same time, bend your neck so that the chin touches or nearly touches your chest and loosen your buttock muscles, allowing room for your back to rise. It should look like a cat stretching its back. Like in Bitilasana, stay in this pose for 15 seconds, breathing normally. Then inhale and return to the starting position. Repeat both the movements about 5 or 6 times before stopping.

If you have a neck injury or back injury, practice these asanas only after consulting your doctor and also in the presence of your yoga trainer. Specifically, for those with serious neck problems, keep your neck in line with your torso.

37. MALASANA (GARLAND POSE)

Malasana is also known as the Garland Pose. It is fundamentally a squatting pose. This asana brings the digestive system back on track and improves metabolism. It reduces belly fat and tones the thighs.

It also stretches the lower back, hips, and groin and is good for your ankles and knees.

To do Malasana, start as you would while doing a squat, but keep your feet near to one another. Now spread your thighs wider than the torso. Exhale and slowly sit down by pushing your buttocks towards the ground. Once your buttocks reach the lowest position, bring your arms in front of your chest, fold them at your elbows and join your palms. Keep breathing naturally. Stay in the pose for 20 - 30 seconds. Then inhale and slowly stand up. If you have a lower back injury or knee injury, refrain from doing this asana.

38. BALASANA

This asana is also known as the Child Pose, as "Bala" translates to "child" in English. Since it is a resting pose, it can be done whenever you feel you want to relax or take a break in between your sessions.

Balasana is an easy yoga pose. It can be done within one to three minutes. It helps to reduce stress and anxiety. Since it stretches the shoulders, hips, and spine, it helps to ease back pain and neck pain. Also, it stimulates digestion and improves bowel movements.

To practice Balasana, kneel down on the floor and sit on your heels. In this position, ensure that your big toes are touching each other. Your knees can be together or hip-width apart, whichever way you find comfortable. Take a deep breath. Now slowly start bending forward such that your forehead touches the floor, as you breathe out. At this point, you can either keep your arms beside you with the palms facing upward or you can stretch your arms in front of you, in a straight line with your knees, palms facing downward. Stay in this position as long as you want and keep breathing actively.

To finish this asana, bring your palms right under your shoulders and press down on the floor. Inhale and slowly lift your upper body. When you return to your initial sitting position (on your heels), exhale. Now, continue breathing naturally and relax.

If you're pregnant, have knee injuries or are suffering from loose motions, you should avoid this asana. In some cases of knee problems, you can ask your yoga teacher for possible modifications. Only if they allow, you can continue doing this asana under proper supervision.

39. SETU BANDHASANA

"Setu" means "bridge" and "Bandha" means "to lock". Setu Bandhasana is called the Bridge Pose. It firms the back muscles, especially in the hips and also stretches the muscles in the neck and chest area. This helps to improve your overall posture. Practicing this asana enhances digestion and blood circulation. It is also beneficial for those diagnosed with thyroid, osteoporosis, asthma, sinusitis, insomnia and high blood pressure.

To practice the Bridge Pose, lie down on the yoga mat flat on your back. Bend your legs at the knees and bring the feet near your buttocks such that the ankles are in line with your knees. Keep your feet hip-width apart. The arms should rest beside you, with your palms facing the floor.

Now, put pressure on your shoulders, arms, knees, and feet. Take a deep breath and slowly raise your back and upper part of your legs (up to your knees) off the mat. You'll notice that without moving your head, your chin touches your chest. Also, your thighs should be parallel to one another and your buttocks firm. Keep breathing. Try to push the torso higher, so that the thighs become parallel to the floor. Stay in the posture for 50 - 60 seconds. Then exhale and slowly lower your back to come out of the pose.

If you're pregnant or have back problems and neck injury, do this asana under your yoga teacher's guidance.

40. BADDHA KONASANA

Baddha Konasana is known by a couple of different names in English. Based on translation, it's called the Bound Angle Pose as "Baddha" means "bound" and "Kona" means "angle" in English. It is also known as the Butterfly Pose because when you move your legs while sitting in this pose, it resembles the flapping action of butterfly wings.

This asana is good for the digestive, urinary and reproductive systems. It improves blood circulation. It should be practiced by pregnant women as it helps in smooth delivery. Baddha Konasana also improves the posture. It stretches the knees and the muscles in the thighs, hips and groin regions. It is said that it can cure flat feet, high blood pressure and asthma.

To do this asana, sit in Dandasana. Next, fold your legs by bending them at the knees. Then bring your feet at the center towards your groin and touch the soles of the feet. Hold the feet tightly with your palms. Keep breathing normally. Ensure that your spine is erect. Now, exhale and lower the knees as much as possible. Start moving your legs up and down at the same time resembling the flapping action of butterfly wings. Slowly increase the speed. Continue for about 1 - 2 minutes. Then exhale and straighten your legs.

If you have sciatica, use a pillow for sitting down and doing this asana. Also, give this asana a miss if you are having your periods or have a knee injury.

41. SUPTA MATSYENDRASANA

Supta Matsyendrasana is called the Supine Twist Pose or the Reclining Twist Pose or the Reclining Lord of the Fish Pose. The last name originates from Supta Matsyendrasana itself as "Supta" means "to lie down" and "Matsyendra" was regarded as the Lord of the Fishes.

Practicing this asana makes the spine more flexible. It stretches the shoulders, chest, hips and the back muscles. It also tones your arms and hips and helps to improve digestion.

Supta Matsyendrasana is done separately on your left and right sides. To practice, start with your right side. Lie down with your back on the mat. Breathe out and slowly extend your arms. Place them on your either sides making a straight line with your shoulders, with the palms facing the floor. Breathe in, lift your right leg and fold it at the knee. Exhale and twist the hip such that your bent right knee crosses over your left thigh. Look to your right, concentrating on your right palm.

Continue breathing normally. With each exhale, twist your hips slightly more and press the left knee down so that it moves closer to the ground. For added support, you can also use your left palm for pressing down your left knee, as long as it feels comfortable. Do this for 20 - 30 seconds and return to the starting position. Then repeat with your left leg.

If you're pregnant, you can use a pillow between your legs. Also, refrain from doing this asana if you have lower back issues.

42. SAVASANA

"Sava" is the Sanskrit for "corpse", so Savasana is also known as the Corpse Pose. It is mandatory to practice this pose at the end of every yoga routine.

Savasana calms your body and mind and releases any kind of stress. It's like a meditation, but by lying down. It enhances memory and concentration power. Savasana also normalizes blood pressure. After a rigorous workout, it helps to restore your energy levels. You can also practice Savasana anytime you feel tired. If you have a busy schedule, practicing it for just 2 – 3 minutes will help you get back to work feeling refreshed.

To do this asana, lie down flat on your yoga mat. Keep your eyes closed. Relax your legs and keep some distance between them. Rest your hands beside you, with palms facing the ceiling. Take long, deep breaths and just focus on yourself for the moment. Focus on each part of your body. Rest like this for about 10 - 15 minutes. Then roll to your left side and slowly sit up. Inhale and exhale a few more times and finally open your eyes.

If you're pregnant, place a bolster under your chest and head for comfort. If your hamstrings or the lower back feel tight, place a bolster or some blankets under your knees.

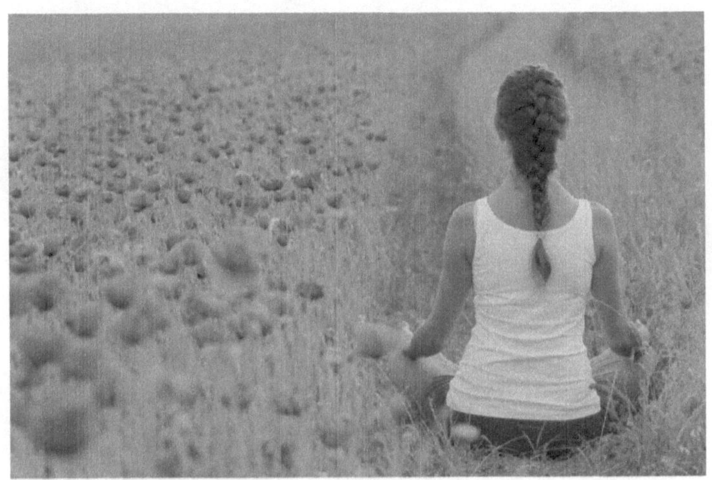

CLEARING MISCONCEPTIONS

Below are some of the most popular misconceptions associated with yoga. Read on to know the truth.

43. FLEXIBILITY IS ESSENTIAL IN YOGA

Only one form of flexibility is important in yoga, and that is mental flexibility. Your physical flexibility is secondary.

People join yoga to become flexible and strong. So how can being flexible be a prerequisite? Think of it this way. Imagine your dream destination. In order to reach that location, you'll have to board some form of transport. Here, flexibility is that "dream destination", while yoga is your transport.

Instead of being a prerequisite, flexibility is actually the end result. So, even if you're as stiff as a machine, yoga will still accept you and will make you flexible. Not only that, yoga will also make you a healthy, balanced individual.

44. YOGA IS ONLY FOR SKINNY PEOPLE

Just like flexibility, your weight is also secondary in yoga.

Specific yoga styles like the Vinyasa Yoga, Hot Yoga, Ashtanga Yoga are great for weight reduction. By practicing yoga regularly, all those fat pockets in your body will slowly start reducing and your muscles will become toned.

45. YOGA DURING PERIODS IS A BIG NO-NO

You can continue to practice yoga during your periods. It will reduce the menstrual cramps and relax your mind. The only kind of poses that you should avoid are the inversions. Remaining other poses are fine, as long as you feel comfortable doing them.

46. YOGA IS JUST FOR YOUNGER PEOPLE

This is a prevailing misconception among the older generation. They think that their reduced mobility coupled with their illnesses such as heart problems, arthritis, knee issues, render them unsuitable for yoga.

But this is completely delusional. Yoga has modifications for each pose depending on the participant's requirements. It allows the use of straps, pillows, blankets, blocks, bolsters etc to support the body as and when needed. Also, yoga instructors are trained professionals who guide you through each step of yoga with patience. With all these options, yoga is definitely accessible for older people as well.

47. YOU'LL HAVE TO CHANGE YOUR FOOD HABITS

Some people believe that if they start doing yoga, they'll have to become vegetarian and/or give up on alcohol and junk food. This is also misleading. Yoga imposes no such restrictions.

Embracing veganism or quitting alcohol and junk food is one's personal choice. You can continue doing yoga with your current food habits.

48. YOGA TEACHERS ARE HEALTH ADVISORS

Yoga teachers surely possess valuable knowledge about human anatomy, but their credentials are very different from that of a certified doctor or a health advisor.

So, next time you have doubts regarding your diet or health supplements or any injuries, consult your doctor first. As per your doctor's advice, ask your yoga instructor to modify your yoga routine.

49. YOGA IS ONLY FOR THE RICH

Even though there are some yoga studios that charge per class, there are also some studios that offer discount packages. These packages usually have 6 - 10 classes depending on the yoga style and are relatively cheaper.

Instead of charging a fixed price, some studios also accept donations. Apart from this, there are community centers that organize yoga classes. If none of these ways work for you, another way to start yoga is by learning via online videos and yoga websites, that provide free, yet useful information.

50. YOGA IS JUST A GENTLE EXERCISE

Yoga has many styles. While some of them are gentle and meditative, others involve rigorous workouts that can leave you red-faced and sweaty. These styles like the Ashtanga Yoga, Hot Yoga or Vinyasa Yoga are physically demanding and require stamina and strength.

Yoga opens the door to all kinds of possibilities. Irrespective of your gender, age, profession and fitness level, you can dive into the awesomeness of yoga. Have confidence in yourself, take the leap of faith and start practicing. Happy Yoga!!

THER HELPFUL RESOURCES:

Free Video Tutorials on Yoga -
https://www.youtube.com/user/yogawithadriene

Free and Paid Video Courses -
https://www.doyouyoga.com/

Further Reading and Video Courses -
https://www.yogajournal.com/

READ OTHER

50 THINGS TO KNOW

BOOKS

50 Things to Know

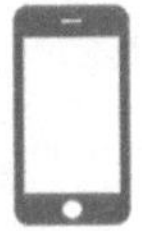

Website: 50thingstoknow.com

Facebook: facebook.com/50thingstoknow

Pinterest: pinterest.com/lbrennec

YouTube: youtube.com/user/50ThingsToKnow

Twitter: twitter.com/50ttk

Mailing List: Join the 50 Things to Know
Mailing List to Learn About New Releases

50 Things to Know

Please leave your honest review of this book on Amazon and Goodreads. We appreciate your positive and constructive feedback. Thank you.